Easy-
My WW I
Complete Cookbook 2024
Easy, And Tasty Family-Friendly WW Recipes for All Ages to Boost Energy

By
Benojir Bhia

By Benojir Bhia
moral right to be identified as the author of this work.

TABLE OF CONTENTS

Baked Frittata with Pesto, Roasted Tomatoes & Goat Cheese

Prep/Cook Time: 55 minutes, Servings 9

Point Values: 5

Ingredients

- 1-2 Tbsp olive oil
- 1 c sweet onions finely chopped
- 2 cloves garlic minced
- 12 large eggs
- ⅓ c pesto prepared
- 1 tsp salt
- ½ tsp pepper
- 1 c roasted tomatoes cut into ½ - inch pieces
- 1 c arugula torn into bite-sized pieces
- 6 oz goat cheese crumbled

Instructions

- Preheat oven to 350 degrees.
- In a medium skillet drizzle olive oil and add onions. Saute onions over medium heat for 5-7 minutes, or until they become translucent.

- Add garlic and saute for an additional 2-3 minutes. Let onions cool until they are close to room temperature.

- In a large bowl combine eggs, pesto, salt and pepper. Whisk to combine.

- Add tomatoes, arugula, goat cheese and onions. Stir until incorporated.

- Spray a 9 x 9-inch square baking dish with non-stick cooking spray.

- Pour mixture into baking dish and bake for 42-48 minutes, or until a toothpick inserted in the center comes out clean.

- Serve with additional pesto, if desired, and enjoy!

Nutrition Info

Calories 201 Calories from Fat 126, Fat 14g, Saturated Fat 5g, Sodium 569mg, Carbohydrates 4g, Sugar 2g, Protein 11g

Spinach Parmesan Baked Eggs Recipe

Prep/Cook Time: 20 Min, Serving: 1

Point Values: 4

Ingredients

- 2 teaspoons olive oil
- 2 garlic cloves minced
- 4 cups baby spinach
- 1/2 cup parmesan cheese fat-free, grated
- 4 eggs
- 1 tomato small, diced small

Instructions

- Preheat oven to 350 degrees. Spray an 8 inch by 8 inch casserole dish with nonstick spray.

- In a large skillet, heat the olive oil on medium heat. Once hot, add the spinach and garlic. Saute until the spinach is wilted. Remove from heat and drain off any excess liquid. Stir in the parmesan cheese and spoon the mixture into an even layer in the casserole dish.

- Create four small divots in the spinach for the eggs. Crack an egg into each divot. Bake for 15 to 20 minutes or until the egg whites are mostly set. Remove from oven and let cool for about 5 minutes then sprinkle with the tomato. Serve and enjoy!

Nutrition Info : Calories: 149kcal, Carbohydrates: 3g, Protein: 12g, Fat: 10g, Saturated Fat: 4g, Cholesterol: 170mg, Sodium: 280mg, Fiber: 1g, Sugar: 1g

Souffle Omelette with Mushrooms

Prep/Cook Time: 25 minutes, Serving: 1

Point Values: 9

Ingredients

- o 1 teaspoon olive oil
- o 1 clove garlic minced
- o 8 ounces mushrooms sliced
- o 1 tablespoon parsley minced
- o 3 large eggs separated
- o 1/4 cup cheddar cheese fat-free, shredded

Instructions

- Over medium heat, in a skillet, warm olive oil and sautè the garlic.
- Add the mushrooms and sautè for 10 minutes. Add the parsley then turn off the heat. Set aside.
- Whisk the egg yolks, until thick. Next, beat the whites until white and frothy. (We used a blender for the egg whites). Fold the whites into the yolks, add cheese, and salt and pepper.
- Spray large skillet with nonstick spray. Pour in the egg mixture then cover. Cook until the top and bottom are set. With the help of a spatula, loosen it carefully. Add the mushrooms to the omelette then carefully fold over. Serve hot.

Nutrition Info : Calories: 329kcal, Carbohydrates: 10g, Protein: 31g, Fat: 19g, Saturated Fat: 6g, Cholesterol: 497mg, Sodium: 375mg, Potassium: 903mg, Fiber: 2g

No-Bake PB & J Energy Bites

Prep/Cook Time: 15 minutes, Servings: 4

Point Values: 3

Ingredients

- 1/2 cup creamy salted peanut butter (or almond, cashew, or sunbutter)
- 1/4 cup maple syrup (or sub finely chopped dates)
- 2 Tbsp vegan protein powder* (optional – just omit if you don't have any)
- 1 1/4 cup gluten-free rolled oats*
- 2 1/2 Tbsp flaxseed meal
- 2 Tbsp chia seeds
- 1/4 cup dried fruit (i.e. dried strawberries, cherries, blueberries, cranberries)

Instructions

- To a large mixing bowl, add peanut butter, maple syrup, protein powder, rolled oats, flaxseed meal, chia seeds, and dried fruit of choice. Mix until well combined. If too dry/crumbly, add more peanut butter or maple syrup. If too sticky or wet, add a little bit more oats or flaxseed meal.

11

- Chill in the refrigerator for 5 minutes. Then scoop out 1 1/2 Tbsp amounts (I like using this scoop) and roll into balls. The "dough" should Servings about 13-14 balls (amount as original recipe is written // adjust if altering batch size).
- Enjoy immediately and store well-sealed leftovers in the refrigerator for 1 week or in the freezer up to 1 month (or more).

Nutrition Info

Calories: 117 Carbohydrates: 13.8 g Protein: 3.6 g Fat: 5.3 g

Instant Pot Cinnamon Apples

Prep/Cook Time: 13 minutes, Servings: 2-4

Point Values: 5

Ingredients

- o 4 medium apples
- o 1 tsp cinnamon
- o 1/8 cup water
- o 1 TBSP sugar, honey, or other sweetener

Instructions

- Peel, core, and chop apples into cubes.
- Place apples and water into your Instant Pot.
- Add cinnamon and sugar and stir well. (If adding honey instead, do that after cooking.)
- Stir well to coat apples with sugar and cinnamon.
- Place lid on and lock.
- Set Instant Pot on Manual for 3 minutes.
- When cooking is complete, a quick release or natural release is fine.
- Serve apples by themselves or with a scoop of vanilla ice cream or pecans!

Nutrition Info

Calories: 203, Carbohydrates: 11g, Protein: 2g, Fat: 14g

Easy Muesli

Point Values: 9

Ingredients

- 160g (2 c) quick cook oats ($0.31 / £0.12)
- 200g (2 c) rolled oats or jumbo oats ($0.38 / £0.50)
- 120g (1½ c) almonds, roughly chopped, or other nuts ($1.80 / £1.01)
- 70g (½ c) sunflower seeds ($0.49 / £0.56)
- 30g (¼ c) pumpkin seeds ($0.41 / £0.24)
- 2 teaspoons Chia seeds, optional ($0.55 / £0.24)
- 200g (1 ¼ c) sultanas or raisins ($1.00 / £0.50)

Instructions

- Preheat the oven to 160°C fan / 180°C / 320°F convection / 356°F.
- Sprinkle the oats in an even layer on a baking tray and place in the preheated oven for 3 minutes. They should start to smell 'oaty' after this time.
- Take the tray out of the oven, stir the oats well, then add the chopped almonds, sunflower seeds and pumpkin seeds, and cook for 5 minutes.
- Remove from the oven and leave to cool on the tray.
- When completely cold, stir in the chia seeds and sultanas or raisins.
- Store in an airtight jar or container for up to 3 weeks.

15

Nutrition Info

Calories: 325kcalCarbohydrates: 45gProtein: 10gFat: 14gSaturated Fat: 1gPolyunsaturated Fat: 5gMonounsaturated Fat: 6gTrans Fat: 0.01gSodium: 8mgPotassium: 455mgFiber: 7gSugar: 1g

Baked Peaches and Cream

Prep/Cook Time: 50 Minutes, Serving: 1

Point Values: 5

Ingredients

- o 4 eggs
- o 1/2 cup milk - use whole or evaporated for a creamier result
- o One 15 ounce container ricotta or cottage cheese - I use Galbani brand, do not use fat free as it contains starches and gum thickeners
- o 1 cup Splenda Granulated - or 1/2 cup Truvia
- o 1½ teaspoons vanilla extract
- o 1/4 teaspoon ground cinnamon
- o 1 teaspoon cornstarch
- o One, 15 ounce can Libby's Splenda sweetened peaches, well drained, wedges split in half

Instructions

- • Preheat oven to 325 degrees. Spray a deep dish pie plate or 2 quart ceramic baking dish with vegetable cooking spray.
- • Combine the the eggs, milk, ricotta, Splenda, vanilla, cinnamon and cornstarch in a blender and puree until very smooth.

- Pour the filling into the baking dish and arrange the peach slices on the custard filling.
- Bake 40 to 45 minutes until the filling is slightly puffed at the edges and is just set meaning it should be firm yet slightly jiggly when you gently move the pie plate from side to side - a little soft in the center is desired.
- Remove from the oven and let cool on a rack. Serve at room temperature or chilled.

Nutrition Info

Calories: 201, Carbohydrates: 13g, Protein: 2g, Fat: 15g

Breakfast Peppers

Prep/Cook Time: 30 Minutes, Serving: 3

Point Values: 4

Ingredients

- o 4 red bell peppers (any color bell pepper works)
- o 16 oz bag frozen, chopped spinach
- o 4 eggs
- o ANYTHING else you want, Bacon,Cheese, Sausage, Onions, Mushrooms, etc...

Instructions

- Preheat oven to 400 degrees. Line the bottom of a baking dish with foil.
- Cut off the top of each pepper. Remove the seeds.
- Place peppers into baking dish and bake for about 15 minutes.
- Meanwhile, defrost the spinach in the microwave. Squeeze the moisture out of the spinach.
- Remove peppers from oven and stuff the bottom 1/2 with cooked spinach.
- Crack an egg into the top 1/2 of each pepper.
- Add any other veggies or cooked meats you'd like.
- Bake for 20 min longer

Nutrition Info : Calories 126, Carbs 11.6, Fat 5.2, Protein 10

Blueberry Cobbler Overnight Oatmeal

Prep/Cook Time: 10 Minutes, Serving: 2

Point Values: 8

Ingredients

- o 3/4 cup Almond milk
- o 1/2 cup Greek yogurt
- o 1 1/2 cup Blueberry
- o 1 cup Old fashioned oats
- o 1/4 cup Protein powder
- o 2 tbs Sweetener of choice
- o 1/4 tsp Salt
- o 1/4 tsp Cinnamon
- o Pinch pinch

Instructions

- In a medium bowl, microwave the blueberries for 30-60 seconds so they pop open. (This will give you more juice and flavor of the berry. Note: if you are using frozen berries, make sure you microwave them until they are thawed). Stir in the rest of ingredients, and divide into two containers. Cover containers and store in the fridge overnight. Top with pecans, additional blueberries, cinnamon, and/or low sugar maple syrup before serving if desired! (Tastes great cold, or microwaved 30-60 seconds)

Nutrition Info : Calories 315, Fat 5 g, Carbohydrate 50 g, Fiber 9 g, Sugar 14 g, Protein 23 g

Sweet Potato and Black Bean Tacos

Prep/Cook Time: 38 minutes, Servings: 5

Point Values: 14

Ingredients

- o 1 1/2 lbs sweet potatoes, peeled and diced into 1/2-inch cubes
- o 4 Tbsp olive oil, divided
- o 1 tsp cumin
- o 1 tsp paprika
- o 1/2 tsp ground coriander
- o 1/4 tsp cayenne pepper (optional)
- o Salt and freshly ground black pepper
- o 1 cup chopped yellow onion, diced
- o 1 1/2 tsp minced garlic
- o 1 (14.5 oz) can black beans, drained and rinsed
- o 1 cup frozen yellow corn, thawed and drained
- o 3 Tbsp honey
- o 3 Tbsp fresh lime juice
- o 2 Tbsp chopped fresh cilantro
- o 10 Corn or flour tortillas
- o Sliced avocado, romaine lettuce, cotija or feta cheese, for serving (optional)

24

Instructions

- Preheat oven to 425 degrees. Line a baking sheet with foil then place sweet potatoes on foil. Drizzle with 3 Tbsp olive oil and toss to evenly coat.

- Sprinkle evenly with cumin, paprika, coriander, cayenne pepper and season lightly with salt and pepper to taste then toss to evenly coat. Bake in preheated oven 15 - 20 minutes until tender, removing from oven and tossing once halfway through baking.

- Meanwhile, in a large skillet, heat remaining 1 Tbsp olive oil over medium-high heat. Once hot add onion and saute until caramelized (golden brown on edges and tender), about 5 - 6 minutes, adding in garlic during last 30 seconds of sauteing.

- Reduce heat to medium-low, add in drained black beans, corn, honey and lime juice. Heat until warmed through. Toss in roasted sweet potatoes and cilantro. Serve over warm tortillas with desired toppings.

Nutrition Info :

Calories 491 Calories from Fat 126, Fat 14g, Saturated Fat 2g, Sodium 282mg, Potassium 949mg, Carbohydrates 86g, Protein 12g24%

Lemon Garlic Shrimp Tostada

Prep/Cook Time: 8 minutes, Servings 4 tostadas

Point Values: 4

Ingredients

- 1/2 pound large uncooked shrimp
- 1/2 teaspoon chopped garlic
- 1/4 cup olive oil
- juice from 1 lemon
- 1/4 teaspoon salt
- 4 baked tostadas
- 1 avocado, diced
- 1 large tomato, diced
- 1 15 ounce can of black beans, cooked (add a pinch of salt to the beans)

Instructions

- In a large bowl add the garlic, olive oil, lemon and salt. Stir with a spoon and then add the shrimp. Cover with saran wrap and refrigerate for at least two hours.
- Place a large skillet on medium heat and add the shrimp. Cook 3-4 minutes on each side or until done. Remove from skillet and set aside.

- To make the tostada top with black beans, avocado, tomatoes and shrimp. Place about 2 teaspoons of shredded monterey jack cheese on top of each tostada.

Nutrition Info

Calories: 199, Sugar: 5g, Fat: 9g, Saturated Fat: 1g, Carbohydrates: 20.4g, Fiber: 8g, Protein: 6g

Grilled Chicken Veggie Bowls

Prep/Cook Time: 1 hr 20 mins, Servings: 8

Point Values: 13

Ingredients :

- o   16 ounces cooked quinoa
- o   16 ounces cooked brown rice
- o   4 cups/32 ounces roasted asparagus chopped
- o   4 cups/32 ounces roasted broccoli florets
- o   4 cups/32 ounces roasted cauliflower florets
- o   32 ounces prepared Grilled Taco Lime Chicken cubed

Optional (would replace any of the vegetables above)

- o   4 cups haricot verts
- o   4 cups roasted brussel sprouts
- o   4 cups charred corn

Instructions

- •   To prepare your bowls, we used 3-cup To Go snack containers. Place 1/4 cup brown rice and 1/4 cup quinoa into each container. Top with a Prep/Cook Time: of 1 1/2 cups of your cooked vegetables. Mix up the type of vegetables for each bowl so you have a variety each day. Add 4 ounces or 1/2 cup of your cubed chicken. We added salsa or hot sauce to season to our liking after we reheated the bowl in the microwave. A low fat dressing would work as well. Store these in the refrigerator and when you are ready microwave until heated through.

Notes

To roast vegetables, place them onto a large baking sheet, drizzle lightly with olive oil, and season with kosher salt and pepper. Cook in oven at 375 degrees until fork tender. Time will vary depending on vegetable.

Nutrition Info

Calories: 662kcal, Carbohydrates: 84g, Protein: 44g

Ingredients

- o 1 Tablespoon olive oil
- o 1 Tablespoon butter
- o 4 Tilapia Fillets cut into 1 inch pieces (you may substitute any other firm, white fish)
- o 2 Tablespoons Zatarains Creole Seasoning
- o 1/4 teaspoon Kosher salt
- o 1/2 head red cabbage coarsely chopped
- o 3 green onions diced
- o 1/2 cup Marzetti Simply Dressed Balsamic Salad Dressing
- o 1 large tomato seeded and diced
- o 2 cups shredded Monterrey Jack cheese
- o 6 small tortillas warmed

Instructions

- In a large skillet, heat olive oil and butter over medium heat, until butter is melted.
- Toss Tilapia fillet pieces with Creole seasoning.
- Add to the skillet and cook over medium heat for 5 minutes, stirring occasionally. Sprinkle with salt.

- While fish is cooking, toss chopped cabbage and onion with Marzetti Simply Dressed Balsamic Salad Dressing. Once combined, add to the skillet with the fish and continue stirring over medium heat until cabbage becomes tender and fish is completely cooked through (approximately 5 minutes).
- Remove from heat.
- Assemble the tortillas with shredded cheese, fish and cabbage mixture, and topped with diced tomatoes. Drizzle with additional Marzetti Simply Dressed Balsamic Salad Dressing, if desired.

Nutrition Info

Calories: 3250, Sugar: 7.1g, Saturated Fat: 8.6g

Low-Carb Slaw

Prep/Cook Time: 25mins, Servings 4

Point Values: 9

Ingredients

- o 1 lb ground beef salt and pepper
- o 2 tablespoons toasted sesame oil
- o 2 garlic cloves, minced
- o 3 green onions, sliced
- o 14 ounces coleslaw mix (if you don't want the carrots use the angel hair cole slaw or just shred up a head of cabbage)
- o 2 tablespoons low sodium soy sauce
- o 1/2 teaspoon sriracha sauce (this will be pretty mild so add to taste or you can use pepper flakes to taste)
- o 1 (1 g) Splenda quick pack
- o 1/2 teaspoon ginger paste (you could also use 1/2 teaspoon fresh minced ginger or ground ginger)
- o 1 teaspoon white vinegar (any kind really)
- o sriracha sauce (to garnish)

Instructions

- • Brown ground beef and season with salt and pepper to taste.
- • Remove from pan and set aside.
- • Heat up sesame oil and sauté garlic, onions, and slaw in sesame oil until cabbage cooked to desired tenderness.

- Stir in the soy sauce, Sriracha sauce, Splenda, ginger and vinegar.
- Add back in hamburger. Mix well and serve!
- Serve with additional Sriracha sauce on the side for people who want to add spice.

Nutrition Info

360 calories; protein 40g; carbohydrates 14g; dietary fiber 2g; sugars 5g; fat 14g; saturated fat 4g; sodium 550mg.

Butternut Squash, Arugula, and Bacon Quiche

Prep/Cook Time: 60 minutes, Servings 12 servings

Point Values: 4

Ingredients

- 1 pie crust, homemade or storebought
- 3 slices bacon, diced
- 2 cups chopped butternut squash
- 1 small white onion, chopped
- 1 clove garlic, minced
- 6 eggs, whisked
- 3/4 cup milk
- 3 Tbsp. flour
- 1/2 tsp. baking powder
- 1/2 tsp. salt
- 1/8 tsp. black pepper
- 3 handfuls fresh arugula, whole or roughly chopped
- 4 ounces crumbled gorgonzola, blue or feta cheese (or any cheese you'd like)

Instructions

- Preheat oven to 350 degrees F.
- Lay prepared pie crust in an ungreased pie plate. Bake for 5 minutes, then set aside.

- Cook bacon in a large saute pan over medium-high heat until crispy, stirring occasionally. Remove bacon with a slotted spoon, leaving grease in pan. Add butternut squash and onion and saute for 8-10 minutes, or until the onions are translucent and the squash is tender. Add garlic and saute for an additional minute. Remove from heat.

- In a separate large bowl, whisk together eggs, flour, baking powder, milk, salt, and black pepper. Stir in the sauteed vegetables, arugula, cheese, and cooked bacon, and stir until well combined.

- Transfer the quiche filling into crust, and use a spoon to smooth the surface. Bake for 45-50 minutes, or until a toothpick inserted comes out clean. Quiche will rise while baking, but should settle back down once you remove it from the oven. Remove from the oven and allow the quiche to rest for at least 5 minutes. Slice and serve warm.

Nutrition Info

300 calories; protein 30g; carbohydrates 12.8g; dietary fiber 3.1g

Stuffed Mini Peppers

Prep/Cook Time: 40 mins, Servings: 50 pieces

Point Values: 1

Ingredients

- o 1 lb mini sweet peppers
- o 2 tbsp extra virgin olive oil
- o salt
- o 10 ounce log goat cheese softened (soft chèvre)
- o 2/3 cup grated parmesan (40g by weight)
- o 1 tbsp minced garlic
- o 2 jalapeños seeded and finely chopped (1/3 cup, measured)
- o 1/4 tsp freshly ground black pepper

Instructions

- Preheat the oven to 425F*.
- De-stem the peppers if desired (I leave them on for aesthetics), then cut each in half. Place in a bowl with the olive oil and 1/4 tsp of salt, and toss well to coat.
- In a large bowl, stir to combine the goat cheese, parmesan, garlic, jalapeno, and black pepper.
- Fill the cut peppers with small spoonfuls of filling. You should have just enough filling to fill the peppers with a

generous amount, coming slightly over the tops of the peppers.

- Roast the peppers for about 20-25 minutes, until the peppers are soft and the cheese is golden on the edges. Enjoy!

Nutrition Info

Calories: 28kcal, Protein: 1g, Fat: 2g, Saturated Fat: 1g, Cholesterol: 3mg,

Better Baked Beans

Ingredients

- 1 (28-ounce) can baked beans
- 1 (16-ounce) can dark red kidney beans, drained
- 1/2 medium onion, finely chopped
- 1/2 cup ketchup
- 2 tablespoons Worcestershire sauce
- 1 tablespoon yellow mustard
- 2 tablespoons apple cider vinegar

Instructions

- Preheat the oven to 350°F and lightly spray a 2-quart baking dish with non-stick cooking spray. . Combine the ingredients in a large bowl and pour the mixture into the baking dish. Bake uncovered for about 45 minutes or until the mixture is bubbly.

Nutrition Info

Calories 420cal , 20.9g Protein, 34g Fat, 2.2g Fiber

Cheese, Spinach & Quinoa Bites

Prep/Cook Time: 55 mins, Servings 24

Point Values: 10

Ingredients

- 2 tsp extra virgin olive oil
- 1 cup uncooked quinoa (Servingss 2 cups cooked)
- 1 cup water
- ½ tsp salt
- 1 tsp extra virgin olive oil
- 1 lb fresh baby spinach (Servingss about 1 cup cooked)
- Pinch of salt
- 3 eggs, lightly beaten
- Salt to taste
- 4 oz Les Petites Fermieres Gouda cheese, cut into 24 cubes
- Cooking Spray

Instructions

TO COOK THE QUINOA

- In a medium saucepan, heat 2 teaspoons of olive oil. Add quinoa and sauté for 3-5 minutes, stirring often, so it's well coated with oil. Add 1 cup water and ½ tsp salt. Bring to a boil, cover and simmer for about 15-20 minutes or until all the water has been absorbed and quinoa is tender, but not mushy. Remove from heat and set aside to cool for 15-20 minutes, then fluff it up with a fork.

- In the meantime, prepare the spinach. Heat 1 teaspoon of olive oil in a large, deep non stick skillet. Add spinach and a pinch of salt and cook over medium heat for 3-4 minutes, until wilted. Set aside to cool
- Preheat oven to 375F. Coat a 24 cup mini muffin pan with cooking spray
- In a large bowl, combine cooked quinoa, cooked spinach, beaten eggs and salt and mix well
- Spoon mixture evenly into the mini muffin pan, so they are ⅔ way full. Tuck a cheese cube in the center of each one
- Bake at 375F for 15 minutes. Serve warm

Nutrition Info

401 calories; protein 50g; carbohydrates 2g; sugars 1g; fat 20g; saturated fat 3g

Canadian Bacon and Pineapple Quesadillas

Prep/Cook Time: 15 min, Servings 4

Point Values: 11

Ingredients

- o 4 (8 to 9-inch) flour tortillas
- o 1/4 to 1/2 cup pizza sauce
- o 1/2 lb. sliced Canadian bacon, cut into small strips
- o 1 (8-oz.) can pineapple tidbits in unsweetened juice, well drained
- o 6 oz. (1 1/2 cups) shredded mozzarella cheese

Instructions

- Place 2 tortillas on ungreased cookie sheet. Spread each with pizza sauce. Top with Canadian bacon, pineapple and 1 cup of the cheese. Top each with remaining tortilla.
- Broil 4 to 6 inches from heat for 1 to 2 minutes. With 2 pancake turners, carefully turn quesadillas over. Sprinkle tops with remaining 1/2 cup cheese.
- Broil an additional 1 to 2 minutes or until cheese is melted and quesadillas are light brown. Cut each into 6 wedges. If desired, serve with additional warm pizza sauce.

Nutrition Info

420 Calories, 16g Prep/Cook Time: Fat, 29g Protein, 40g Prep/Cook Time: Carbohydrate, 8g Sugars

41

Chicken Avocado Burger

Prep/Cook Time: 15 Minutes, Serving: 4

Point Values: 6

Ingredients

- o 1 lb ground chicken (or turkey)
- o 1/2 ripe avocado, cubed
- o 1/2 cup grated parmesan cheese
- o 1 clove garlic, pressed
- o 1/4 tsp each salt and pepper

Instructions

- Cut the avocado half into chunks. Toss with parmesan cheese and garlic.
- Fold the mixture into the ground chicken being cautious not to mash the avocado.
- Form the mixture into 4 burger patties (or 6 smaller patties). Heat a grill pan on the stovetop to medium and grill on each side for about 5 minutes. Check the temperature is at 165F before serving.

Nutrition Info

Calories: 260kcal, Carbohydrates: 5g, Protein: 24g, Fat: 12g, Saturated Fat: 5g, Trans Fat: 1g

Easy Italian Meatloaf

Prep/Cook Time: 60 Minutes, Serving: 6

Point Values: 7

Ingredients

- 1 lb lean ground beef
- 1/2 cup spaghetti sauce, divided
- 1/2 cup grated parmesan cheese, divided
- 1/4 cup shredded 2% mozzarella cheese
- 1/4 cup finely chopped onion
- 1 egg, lightly beaten
- 1 tsp Italian seasoning

Instructions

- Preheat oven to 375°F. Mix meat, 1/4 cup of the spaghetti sauce, grated parmesan cheese, 1/4 cup of the shredded cheese, onion, egg and seasoning.
- Shape into loaf in 12x8-inch baking dish. Top with remaining 1/4 cup spaghetti sauce and remaining cheese.
- Bake 40 to 45 minutes or until cooked through (160°F). *Tip: speed up cooking time by 10-15 minutes by making two smaller loaves

Nutrition Info

Calories: 257kcal, Carbohydrates: 3g, Protein: 31g, Fat: 13g, Saturated Fat: 4g, Trans Fat: 1g

Garlic & Basil Shrimp with Tomatoes

Prep/Cook Time: 20 Minutes, Serving: 4

Point Values: 4

Ingredients

o 1 lb medium frozen shrimp

o 1 (14.5 oz) can Muir Glen® Diced Tomatoes

o 2 tbsp Light Italian Dressing

o 2 tbsp grated parmesan cheese

o 2 tbsp fresh chopped basil

Instructions

- Thaw shrimp by running under cold water and remove tails. Place in a large bowl and add Italian dressing. Let marinade while pan heats.

- Heat a non-stick pan to medium and spray with olive oil or cooking spray. Add shrimp and cook about 5 minutes, stirring on occasion.

- Add tomatoes; stir a few more times and cook about 2-3 minutes.

- Remove from heat and scoop onto serving plates. Add grated parmesan cheese and shaved parmesan cheese.

Nutrition Info

Calories: 110kcal, Carbohydrates: 6g, Protein: 30g, Fat: 1g, Saturated Fat: 1g, Trans Fat: 1g, Cholesterol: 288mg, Sodium: 989mg

Mini Bariatric Sized Meatloaf

Prep/Cook Time: 20 Minutes, Serving: 4

Point Values: 8

Ingredients

- 1 lb 93% lean ground beef
- 1 1/4 tsp salt
- 1/4 tsp black pepper
- 1/2 cup green bell pepper finely diced
- 1/2 cup onion, finely chopped
- 1 egg slightly beaten or 1/2 cup egg substitute
- 1/2 cup grated parmesan cheese
- 8 oz petite diced tomatoes
- 2 tbsp low sugar ketchup or try it with bbq sauce

Instructions

- Preheat over to 375 degrees. Lightly spray muffin tins with cooking spray.
- Add ground beef, salt, pepper, onion, bell pepper, parmesan cheese and egg to a bowl.
- Add diced tomatoes and part of juice until the consistency you want – not moist enough to fall apart.
- Using clean hands mix ingredients together.
- Divide mixture into muffin pans and top with ketchup or bbq sauce.

- Bake for 30-35 minutes; let cool before serving.

Nutrition Info

Calories: 331kcal, Carbohydrates: 8g, Protein: 38g, Fat: 15g, Saturated Fat: 7g

Hamburger Salad

Prep/Cook Time: 20 Minutes, Serving: 4

Point Values: 6

Ingredients

- o 1 lb 93% lean ground beef
- o pinch each salt & pepper
- o 1 tbsp burger seasoning of choice
- o 8 oz mixed greens
- o 4 slices turkey bacon, cooked and diced
- o 1 tbsp diced pickle slices as desired
- o 1 tsp each mustard & low sugar ketchup as desired

Instructions

- Heat a grill pan to medium high on the stovetop. Cover lightly with cooking spray.
- Form ground beef into four patties, sprinkling both sides with salt and pepper.
- Brown both sides of patties, about 3 minutes per side. Use a spatula to break the burger to smaller chunks to continue cooking faster. Sprinkle generously with seasoning of choice for added flavor.
- Meanwhile, layer chopped lettuce on a plate or in a bowl. Add turkey bacon. Squirt mustard and ketchup as

desired. Dice pickle slices up if desired. Once ground beef is cooked, add to salad.

Nutrition Info

200 calories; protein 10g; carbohydrates 11g; dietary fiber 3.4g; sugars 4g; fat 14g; saturated fat 5.4g

Sun Dried Tomato & Feta Chicken Bake

Prep/Cook Time: 35 Minutes, Serving: 4

Point Values: 4

Ingredients

- 1 lb boneless, skinless chicken breast
- 3 tbsp sun dried tomatoes, rinsed well and chopped
- 3 cloves garlic, pressed or minced
- 2 tbsp dried basil
- 1/4 tsp each salt and pepper
- 1/2 cup feta cheese crumbles (optional)

Instructions

- Preheat oven to 375.
- Place chicken in the bottom of a baking dish and toss with basil, salt, pepper and garlic to coat.
- Spread a layer of sun-dried tomatoes over each chicken breast. Cover dish with a piece of foil.
- Bake for 20 minutes then remove foil and bake for another 15 minutes or until chicken is cooked through (165F).
- Remove from oven and add feta to each chicken breast, if using. Let rest two minutes before serving.

Nutrition Info

Calories: 160kcal, Carbohydrates: 3g, Protein: 27g, Fat: 4g, Saturated Fat: 4g, Trans Fat: 1g, Cholesterol: 89mg

Chicken Enchilada Stuffed Zucchini Boats

Prep/Cook Time: 1 hr, Servings 4 servings

Point Values: 6

Ingredients

For the enchilada sauce:

- olive oil spray ,
- 2 garlic cloves, minced
- 1 or 2 tbsp chipotle chile in adobo sauce, more if you like it spicy
- 1-1/2 cups tomato sauce
- 1/2 tsp chipotle chili powder
- 1/2 tsp ground cumin
- 2/3 cup fat-free low-sodium chicken broth
- kosher salt and fresh pepper to taste

For the zucchini boats:

- 4 about 32 oz Prep/Cook Time: medium zucchini
- 1 tsp oil
- 1/2 cup green onions, chopped
- 3 cloves garlic, crushed
- 1/2 cup diced green bell pepper
- 1/4 cup chopped cilantro, plus more for garnish
- 8 oz cooked shredded chicken breast

- o 1 tsp cumin
- o 1/2 tsp dried oregano
- o 1/2 tsp chipotle chili powder
- o 3 tbsp water or chicken broth
- o 1 tbsp tomato paste
- o salt and pepper to taste

For the Topping:

- o 3/4 cup reduced fat shredded sharp cheddar
- o cilantro for garnish

Instructions

For the enchilada sauce:

- In a medium saucepan, spray oil and sauté garlic.
- Add chipotle chiles, chili powder, cumin, chicken broth, tomato sauce, salt and pepper and bring to a boil.
- Reduce the heat to low and simmer for 5-10 minutes. Set aside until ready to use.

Meanwhile For the Zucchini Boats:

- Preheat oven to 400°F.

- Cut zucchini in half lengthwise and using a small spoon or melon baller, scoop out flesh, leaving 1/4" thick.

- Chop the scooped out flesh of the zucchini in small pieces and set aside.

- In a large saute pan, heat oil and add onion, garlic and bell pepper.

- Cook on medium-low heat for about 2-3 minutes, until tender.

- Add chopped zucchini and cilantro; season with salt and pepper and cook about 4 minutes.

- Add the cumin, oregano, chili powder, water, and tomato paste and cook a few more minutes, then add in chicken; mix and cook 3 more minutes.

- Place 1/4 cup of the enchilada sauce on the bottom of a large (or 2 small) baking dish, and place zucchini halves cut side up.

- Using a spoon, fill each hollowed zucchini with 1/3 cup chicken mixture, pressing firmly.

- Top each with 2 tablespoons of enchilada sauce, and 1 1/2 tablespoons each of shredded cheese.

- Cover with foil and bake 35 minutes until cheese is melted and zucchini is tender.

- Top with scallions and cilantro for garnish and serve with Greek yogurt or sour cream, if desired.

Nutrition Info

Calories: 232 kcal, Carbohydrates: 22 g, Protein: 24 g, Fat: 7 g, Cholesterol: 44 mg, Sodium: 820 mg, Fiber: 6 g, Sugar: 9 g

Grilled Honey Mustard Chicken

Point Values: 10

Ingredients

- o 1/2 cup of any whole grain mustard
- o 1/2 cup of honey
- o Juice of ½ a lemon
- o 1 garlic clove smashed and minced
- o 1/2 teaspoon paprika
- o 1/2 teaspoon salt
- o 1/4 teaspoon cayenne pepper
- o 1/4 teaspoon red pepper flakes
- o 4 boneless skinless chicken breasts

Instructions

- Whisk all ingredients in a small bowl. Reserve 4 tablespoons of sauce and then pour the remaining honey mustard mixture over the chicken, toss and cover with plastic wrap and let it sit for about 30-45 minutes at room temperature.

- Preheat the grill on medium-medium high heat, grill chicken for about 6 to 7 minutes per side or until chicken is done.

- Pour the reserved honey-mustard sauce over chicken and let rest under foil for about 5 minutes. Serve.

Nutrition Info

Calories 410kcal Carbohydrates37g Protein50g Fat7g

Slow Cooker Sloppy Joe Bowl

Prep/Cook Time: 6 hours 10 minutes, Servings: 4 servings

Point Values: 5

Ingredients

- o 1 lb 97% lean ground beef
- o 1 small red onion, diced
- o 1 (10.75 oz) can diced tomatoes
- o 2 tbsp worcestershire sauce
- o 1/2 cup ketchup (under 8 grams sugar)

Instructions

- Brown the ground beef in a skillet, adding a pinch of salt and pepper to season, and drain after cooking. Move to the bottom of a slow cooker.
- Add all the other ingredients: red onion, diced tomatoes, Worcestershire sauce and ketchup. Stir to combine.
- Cook on low for 6 hours.
- Serve in a bowl with cooked veggies such as a steamer bag of cauliflower, broccoli and carrots.

Nutrition Info

Calories: 208kcal, Carbohydrates: 9g, Protein: 23g, Fat: 8g, Saturated Fat: 5g, Trans Fat: 1g, Cholesterol: 74mg, Sodium: 535mg, Potassium: 473mg, Fiber: 1g

Prep/Cook Time: 20 Minutes, Serving: 6

Point Values: 4

Ingredients

- o 1 lb 93% lean ground beef
- o 1/4 tsp each salt and pepper
- o 1/4 avocado, sliced
- o 1 tbsp chopped cilantro
- o 3 strips maple turkey bacon regular okay if no maple available
- o 3 slices reduced fat pepperjack cheese

Instructions

- Form the ground beef into 4 patties. Using either a grill or grill pan, heat to medium. Sprinkle salt and pepper on each side of the patty and grill. Flip once at the 5 minute mark and grill another 5 minutes.
- Meanwhile, cook the turkey bacon in a separate skillet for 4 minutes, turning once. Slice the avocado and chop the cilantro.
- Once all the ingredients are ready, assemble burger with toppings. Place the burger on the plate and top with half slice of cheese, half slice of turkey bacon, one slice avocado and cilantro in that order.

Nutrition Info

Calories: 175kcal, Carbohydrates: 2g, Protein: 21g, Fat: 9g, Saturated Fat: 4g, Trans Fat: 1g, Cholesterol: 57mg, Sodium: 215mg, Potassium: 313mg, Fiber: 1g

Peruvian Soup

Prep/Cook Time: 17 minutes, Servings 4

Point Values: 3

Ingredients

- o   1 poblano pepper; de-seeded and diced
- o   1 white onion; diced
- o   2 tablespoons minced garlic
- o   1 serrano; diced
- o   4 cups chicken stock
- o   1 whole rotisserie chicken; skin removed
- o   10 mini yellow potatoes; quartered
- o   2 cups frozen peas and carrots
- o   1 bundle fresh cilantro leaves
- o   1 lime; juiced
- o   2 teaspoons salt
- o   2 teaspoons pepper
- o   water

Instructions

- Place diced onion, poblano pepper, serrano pepper, and garlic into the blender. Add two cups chicken broth and puree.

- Pour mixture into the instant pot. Shred chicken from rotisserie removing skin and place chicken into the instant pot.

- Pour in the remaining chicken broth and water. Quarter potatoes and add to the instant pot. Place lid on instant pot and set pressure valve to close.

- Set to high pressure for 8 minutes. Once the instant pot stops counting quick release pressure.

- Turn instant pot to "sauté" and add in peas and carrots. Cook for about 3 minutes until carrots are tender.

- To the blender add a 1/3 cup water, lime juice, and cilantro bundle. Blend well. Pour this while stirring into the soup. Add salt and pepper.

- Stir well and turn off "sauté" mode. Your soup is now ready to serve.

Nutrition Info

Calories: 690Prep/Cook Time: Fat: 10gSaturated Fat: 3gTrans Fat: 0g

Asparagus Soup

Point Values: 2

Ingredients

- o 2 Tablespoons Olive Oil
- o 1 lb Fresh Asparagus, (woody ends removed, chopped into 3" pieces)
- o 1 White Onion
- o 2 Garlic Cloves
- o 4 Cups Vegetable Stock or Vegetable Broth
- o 2 Starchy Potatoes (peeled and chopped)
- o 1 Bay Leaf
- o Salt & Black Pepper

Instructions

Prepare Vegetables

- Peel and chop your potatoes and onion. Remove the woody ends from your asparagus spears. Be sure to leave the asparagus tips and chop each asparagus spear into thirds.
- Set your Instant Pot to sauté setting and add your olive oil. Add potatoes, onions and chopped asparagus spears to the pot. Add garlic cloves and saute for two minutes.
- Turn off the sauté function and add the vegetable broth and bay leaf.

- Stir and scrape the bottom of the pot with a wooden spoon to ensure no pieces of garlic, onion or asparagus are stuck to the bottom of the inner pot.

- Close the Instant Pot Lid. Set the Instant Pot to pressure cook or manual setting and cook your soup for 15 minutes under high pressure.

- Once the pressure cooking time has been completed, allow the pressure to naturally release for 10 minutes then quickly release the remaining pressure.

- A quick release could result in the liquid spewing out the vent. So it is better to perform a natural release.

- Once all the pressure has been released, open the Instant Pot lid and remove the bay leaf.

- Transfer the soup mixture to a blender or food processor and blend into a nice creamy texture.

- Alternatively, you can use an immersion blender and blend the asparagus soup directly in the Instant Pot. This is a quick, easy and less messy way to blend your asparagus soup.

- Season your Instant Pot Asparagus Soup. Add salt and pepper and garnish with fresh herbs.

- There you have it, a fresh-tasting, healthy vegan asparagus soup recipe that the whole family can enjoy!

Nutrition Info :

Calories: 193Prep/Cook Time: Fat: 8gSaturated Fat: 1gTrans Fat: 0gUnsaturated Fat: 6g

Cauliflower Soup with Parmesan

Prep/Cook Time: 30 minutes, Servings 6

Point Values: 3

Ingredients

- o 2 – 3 pounds of Cauliflower florets
- o 4 teaspoons of minced garlic
- o 1 sweet onion – chopped
- o 6 cups of chicken broth
- o 1 carton of sour cream – 4 – 6 ounces
- o 1 Tablespoon of coarse ground garlic salt
- o 1 teaspoon of seasoned pepper
- o 1 jar of Sun Dried Tomatoes
- o Crumbled bacon – for topping
- o 1 bunch of green onions – washed and finely chopped
- o 2 tubs of Shredded Parmesan cheese – 16 ounces each

Instructions

- First, line a cookie sheet with Parchment paper (or use silpat) and drop Tablespoons of Parmesan cheese onto the Parchment paper, about 2 inches apart, in little bunches, and sprinkle with Italian seasoning.
- Place the cookie sheet in the oven at 350 degrees for about 10 – 15 minutes, or until the Parmesan starts to turn golden brown.

- Remove the cookie sheet from the oven, and let cool. These are the Parmesan croutons for the soup, so make as many as you like, depending on how many you're serving. (I made 2 croutons per bowl of soup served).

- Next, rinse the Cauliflower, and break it into florets. Chop the florets into small pieces. Chop the sweet onion, and place the Cauliflower florets, onion, minced garlic, chicken broth, garlic salt, and seasoned pepper in the Instant Pot.

- Stir well, and place the lid on the Instant Pot, until it beeps and locks. Make sure the pressure valve is set to SEALING, and press the Manual button, and set the time for 10 minutes.

- Let the Instant Pot build the pressure, cook the soup, and then naturally release the pressure. When the IP beeps, and goes to the OFF setting, make sure the FLOAT VALVE is down, and all the pressure has been released, and then remove the lid.

- Stir the soup, and using an immersion blender, blend the soup into a smooth creamy mixture. Add the sour cream, and about 8 ounces of Parmesan cheese, and stir well.

- When ready to serve ladle the soup into bowls, place two of the Parmesan croutons in each bowl, and drizzle a little oil from the Sun dried Tomatoes, on to the top of the soup. Top with crumbled bacon, and green onions.

Nutrition Info

Calories: 439Prep/Cook Time: Fat: 25gSaturated Fat: 14gTrans Fat: 0gUnsaturated Fat: 9gCholesterol: 66mgSodium: 3136mg

Thai Chicken Soup

Prep/Cook Time: 21 minutes, Servings 4-5

Point Values: 17

Ingredients

- 2 Tbsp avocado oil
- 1 Onion, diced
- 1 tbsp garlic, minced
- 2 Tbsp Ginger paste
- 1 Tbsp Lemongrass paste
- 2 Red peppers, thinly sliced
- 8 ounces Sliced Baby Bella mushrooms
- 6 Boneless skinless chicken thighs cut into cubes
- 3 Cups Chicken Broth
- 1 14 oz Can coconut milk, full fat
- 3 Tbsp Fish sauce
- 3 Tbsp Lime juice
- 1 Tbsp Soy sauce
- 2 tsp Thai red curry paste
- Fresh cilantro for garnish

Instructions

- Heat a 6 or 8 quart Instant Pot, using the sauté function. Add oil, chicken, red peppers, and onions, and sauté 2-3 minutes.

- Add the mushrooms, and cook for 2 minutes. Add lemon grass paste, ginger paste, curry paste, fish sauce, soy sauce and stir. Allow to sit for 2 minutes.

- Add the broth and stir. Close the lid, seal the pressure valve, and set on manual/high for 4 minutes.

- Once the time is up, let the pressure release naturally for 5-10 minutes, then flip the valve to release the remaining pressure. Remove the top carefully. Add lime juice, coconut milk and stir to combine.

- Serve the soup and garnish Thai basil.

Nutrition Info

Calories: 623Prep/Cook Time: Fat: 44gSaturated Fat: 24gTrans Fat: 0gUnsaturated Fat: 18gCholesterol: 209mgSodium: 2346mgCarbohydrates: 18gFiber: 3gSugar: 7gProtein: 47g

Vegan Cherry Chocolate Chip Ice Cream

Prep/Cook Time: 3 hours, 14 minutes, 59 seconds,

Point Values:

Ingredients

- 2 cups cherries, fresh
- 1/2 banana
- 1/2 cup unsweetened almond milk
- 3 tablespoons dairy-free chocolate chips

Instructions

- Wash and dry the cherries, and remove all the pits. Place in a freezer bag or glass container, and freeze for at least three hours. If you don't have the time, you can use frozen cherries.
- Peel a banana, and place half in the freezer.
- Pour 1/4 cup of the almond milk into ice cube trays (save the other 1/4 cup), and freeze those as well, for at least three hours.
- Place the frozen cherries, half a frozen banana, the almond-milk ice cubes, and 1/4 cup almond milk in a

food processor, and process until completely smooth, several minutes.

- Stir in chocolate chips, and enjoy immediately!

Nutrition Info

Calories 126 calories

Prep/Cook Time: 3 Minutes, Serving: 2

Point Values: 6

Ingredients

- o 1 tablespoons cocoa powder, unsweeted
- o 2 packets truvia (may substitute for other sweeteners)
- o 2 tablespoons all purpose flour (may substitute for Almond Flour)
- o 3 tablespoons almond milk (may substitute for regular milk or yogurt)

Instructions

- Place all ingredients in a microwave safe mug. Mix with a fork or small whisk
- Microwave on high for 60 seconds
- Enjoy!

Nutrition Info

Calories 97, fat 25.1g; saturated fat 5g

Triple Berry Cobbler

Prep/Cook Time: 3 hrs 45 mins, Servings: 12

Point Values: 4

Ingredients

Nonstick cooking spray

- o 1 14 ounce package frozen loose-pack mixed berries
- o 1 21 ounce can blueberry pie filling
- o 2 tablespoon sugar
- o 1 6.5 ounce package blueberry muffin mix
- o ⅓ cup water
- o 2 tablespoon vegetable oil
- o Plain Greek yogurt (optional)
- o Honey (optional)

Instructions

- Lightly coat a 3 1/2- or 4-quart slow cooker with cooking spray; set aside.
- In cooker combine frozen berries, pie filling, and sugar.
- Cover and cook on low-heat setting for 3 hours. Turn cooker to high-heat setting. In a medium bowl combine muffin mix, the water, and oil; stir just until combined. Spoon muffin mixture over berry mixture.
- Cover and cook for 1 hour more or until a wooden toothpick inserted into center of muffin mixture comes out clean. Turn off cooker. If possible, remove crockery

liner from cooker. Cool, uncovered, for 30 to 45 minutes on wire rack before serving.

- If desired, serve with yogurt and honey.

Nutrition Info

162 Calories, 4g Fat, 31g Carbs, 1g Protein

Valentine Berry Breakfast Smoothie

Prep Time 10 minutes, Servings 1

Point Values: 8

Ingredients

- o 1 cup unsweetened vanilla almond milk
- o ⅓ cup plain Greek yogurt
- o 1 scoop Bariatric Fusion Vanilla High Protein Meal Replacement
- o 1 scoop Bariatric Fusion Strawberry High Protein Meal Replacement
- o ¼ cup blueberries
- o ¼ cup raspberries
- o 1 tbsp hemp hearts

Instructions

- • Combine all ingredients in a blender. Process until rich and creamy, then serve cold and enjoy!
- • Store leftovers in the refrigerator in an airtight container. To re-serve, add ice, re-blend, and consume within 24 hours.

Nutrition Info

Calories 331, Fat 10 grams, Carbs 24 grams, Fiber 7.5 grams, Sugar 10 grams, Protein 40 grams

Mango Peach Smoothie

Prep/Cook Time: 5 Minutes, Serving: 1

Point Values: 3

Ingredients

- o 1 cup nonfat Greek Style Yogurt
- o ½ cup Skim Milk
- o ½ cup frozen Peaches
- o ½ cup frozen Mango
- o 1 cup ice

Instructions

- In a blender add yogurt and frozen fruit. Add in milk. Top with ice. Mix until smooth. Enjoy immediately.

Nutrition Info

240 calories; protein 17.2g; carbohydrates 13.7g

Peanut Butter Smoothie

Prep/Cook Time: 10 Minutes, Serving: 2

Point Values: 3

Ingredients:

- o 1 small frozen banana
- o 400ml calci trim milk
- o 1 tbsp protein powder (I used NZ Protein's peanut butter pea protein)
- o 1 tbsp peanut butter
- o 1 tsp cinnamon
- o Cocoa powder for dusting (optional)

Instructions

- Allow the banana to defrost on the bench for 10 minutes before peeling and adding into a blender
- Add the remaining ingredients except for the cocoa and blitz until well combined
- Pour into two glasses and dust with extra cocoa if you would like

Nutrition Info

170 calories; protein 24.1g; carbohydrates 7.2g

Made in the USA
Monee, IL
28 June 2024